Treat Depression

NATURALLY

7 Life Essences that will help you Fight Depression

By

DeNise Renee Muhammad

Table of Contents

Acknowledgements

In the Name of Allah the Beneficent the Merciful. I bear witness there is no God but Allah and that Muhammad is his Messenger.

I would like to first and foremost thank Allah (God) for blessing me with gifts, skills and talents. I also thank my Business Coach, Dawniel Winningham for allowing God to use her to place the idea in my mind to even write a book when I didn't even know that it was in me! Last but certainly not least, I thank my business partner and friend, Brother Sean Ali, for inspiring me to finish my book. He gave me that push when I needed it to get it done! May Allah continue to bless us all to make unlimited progress!

Treat Depression

NATURALLY

7 Life Essences that will help you Fight Depression

Introduction

According to the Anxiety and Depression Association of America, depression is a condition that affects more than 15 million American adults, or about 6.7 percent of the United States population age 18 or older in a given year. The National Network of Depression Centers (NNDC) states that depression is the leading cause of disability in the United States among people ages 15-44. The NNDC also states that depression ranks among the Top 3 workplace issues in the US, along with family crisis and stress.

Some of the symptoms of depression include: sadness, irritability, lethargy, insomnia, loss of interest in everyday activities, and just general unhappiness. My intention for writing this book, is to give you a natural way to support a healthy mental state with LIFE Essences aka essential oils, which are not actually oils they are the life essence of a plant. I will also show you how to use them. Some anti-depressant drugs on the market have been found by scientists to actually worsen mental health issues. Essential oils are the oldest plant based medicinal known to man that have absolutely no side effects. Before you consider taking anti-depressants, open your mind to a natural way to support your mental well-being.

Powerful Influence of Aromas

"The fragrance of an essential oil can directly affect everything from your emotional state to your lifespan. The specific mechanics of the sense of smell are still being explored by scientists but have been described as working like a lock and key or an odor molecule fitting a specific receptor site.

When a fragrance is inhaled, the airborne odor molecules travel up the nostrils to the olfactory epithelium, which is only about 1 square inch of the nasal cavity, olfactory receptor cells are triggered and send an impulse to the olfactory bulb," as stated in the Life Science Publishing Essential Oils Pocket Reference Guide. Aromatherapy is so powerful that you can inhale it directly from the bottle to help you fight food cravings. If you are practicing eating one meal a day or also known as intermittent fasting, and you start to feel hungry before it's time for you to eat, you can inhale peppermint oil and it will curb your appetite.

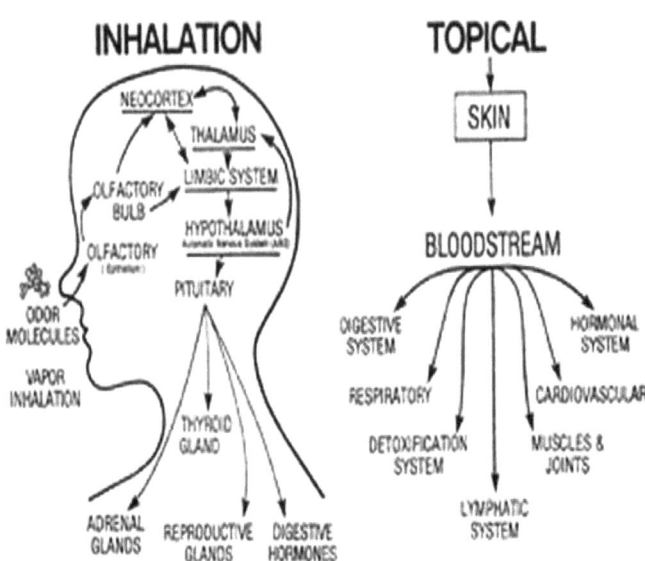

Chapter 1

Lemon Essential Oil

Lemon essential oil has fantastic energizing properties. It has a stimulant like effect on the brain and energizing effect on the body, which in turn creates an energizing and mood enhancing effect. Limonene is a key constituent in the lemon essential oil. According to WebMD, "Limonene is a chemical found in the peels of citrus fruits and in other plants. It is used to make medicine.

Limonene is used to promote weight loss, prevent cancer, treat cancer, and treat bronchitis." Life Science Publishing Essential Oils Pocket Reference Guide states, lemon essential oil promotes clarity of thought and purpose with a fragrance that is invigorating, enhancing, and warming. Just from inhaling lemon oil, your spirits will immediately be lifted. It has a sweet lemony aroma that just makes me smile. It is a staple in my home and one of my favorite oils by far. There are so many more benefits to this oil but for the purpose of this book I'll stick to how it can help you with depression.

How to Use Lemon Essential Oil to treat Depression:

- Take three drops underneath the tongue in the morning and at night. This is the quickest way for the oil to absorb in the blood stream.
- Take two to three drops of lemon in 8 ounces if water. Drink this first thing in the morning to start your day. You can also drink this as a midday pick-me-up.

- Diffuse 5-10 drops or steam vaporize throughout the day. Constant exposure to the vapors alleviates both emotional and physical symptoms of depression.
- Lemon oil can be used topically in its undiluted form. You can add one to two drops to the bridge of the nose, behind the ears, reflex points, or the bottom of your feet.
- As a quick fix, put a drop or two in the palm of your hands, rub them together and then cup your hands around the nose and mouth then breathe in deeply.

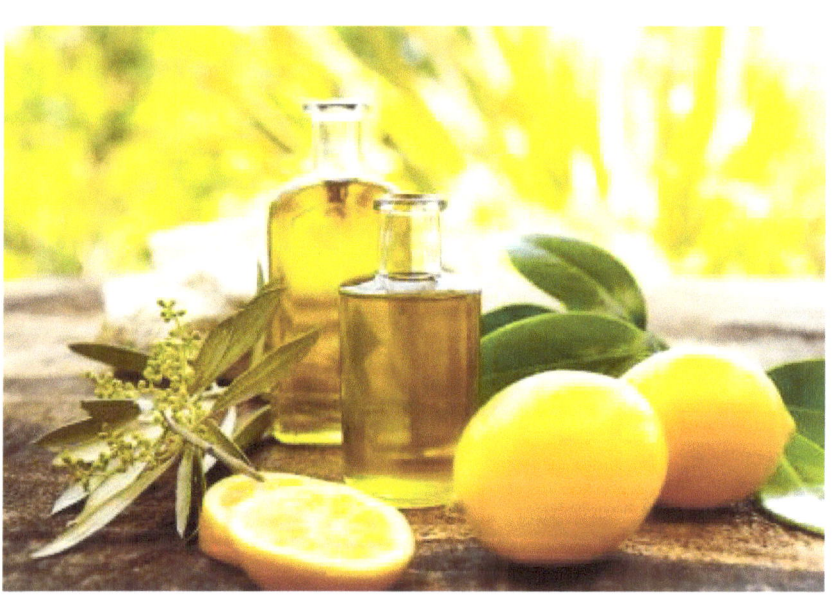

Chapter 2

Orange Essential Oil

The next oil that we have that helps with fighting depression is Orange Essential Oil. The very smell of orange essential oil reminds me of happy moments from my childhood. This is why this oil is frequently used in aromatherapy. It creates a happy, relaxed feeling and works as a mood lifter. Orange essential oil is perfect for people who suffer with depression and anxiety. Not to mention the plethora of other health benefits of using orange essential oil. It is antitumor, a relaxant, anticoagulant, and a circulatory stimulant. According to the Essential Oils Pocket Reference Guide, orange essential oil is "rich in limonene, which has been extensively studied over 50 clinical studies for its ability to combat tumor growth."

How to use Orange Essential Oil to fight Depression:

- Take two to three drops of orange oil in 8 ounces if water. Drink this first thing in the morning to start your day. You can also drink this as a midday pick-me-up.
- Diffuse 5-10 drops or steam vaporize throughout the day. Constant exposure to the vapors alleviates both emotional and physical symptoms of depression.
- Orange oil can be used topically in its undiluted form. You can add one to two drops to the bridge of the nose, behind the ears, reflex points, or the bottom of your feet. You can also dilute it with a carrier oil, such as coconut oil, and rub it on your skin or pulse points.

- As a quick fix, put a drop or two in the palm of your hands, rub them together and then cup your hands around the nose and mouth then breathe in deeply.

As a side note, "diffusing or directly inhaling essential oils can have an immediate, positive impact on mood. Olfaction (smell) is the only sense that can have direct effects on the limbic region of the brain. Studies at the University of Vienna have shown that some essential oils and their primary constituents (cineole) can stimulate blood flow and activity in the emotional regions of the brain" stated in the Essential Oils Pocket Reference Guide.

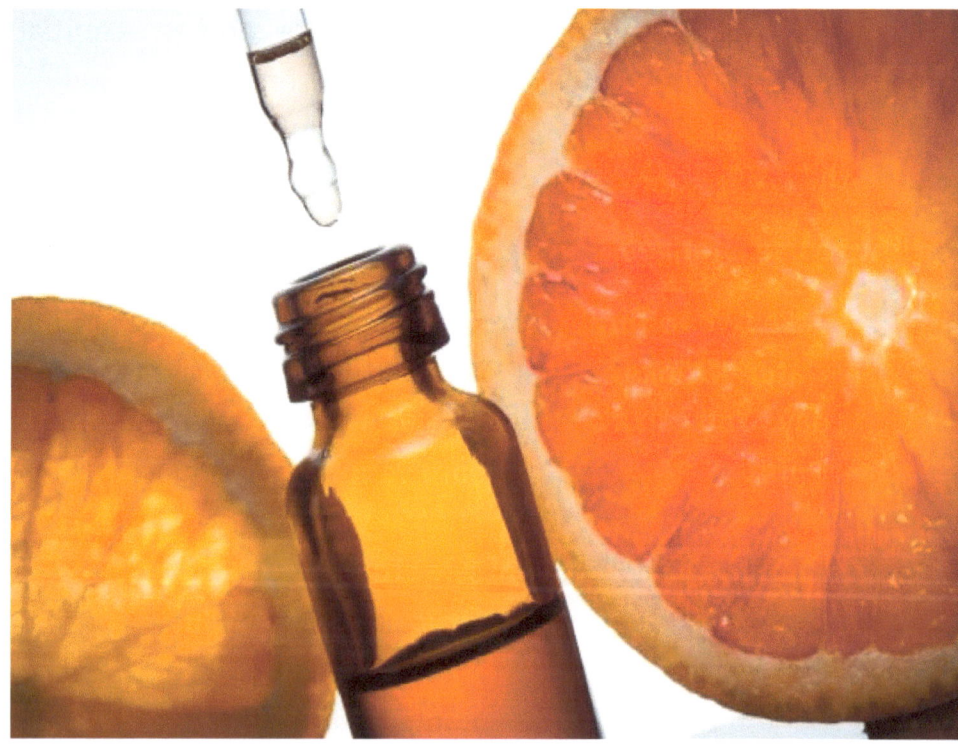

Chapter 3

Lavender Essential Oil

Lavender is a flowering plant from the mint family. It is native to the Old World and is found from Cape Verde and the Canary Islands, Europe across to northern and eastern Africa, the Mediterranean, southwest Asia to southeast India.

Lavender has antiseptic, anti-inflammatory properties and is a relaxant. Lavender essential oil is one of my absolute favorites! It is a staple in my house. I love the way it smells and the way it makes me feel calm and relaxed. This is another oil that is good to help you fight depression naturally. Lavender essential oil is well known for helping you relax and fall asleep; however, it is also great for depression.

The fragrant influence of lavender is that it is calming, relaxing, and balancing, both physically and emotionally. Lavender has been documented to improve concentration and mental acuity. According to the Essential Oils Pocket Reference guide, the "University of Miami researchers found that inhalation of lavender oil increased beta waves in the brain, suggesting heightened relaxation. It also reduced depression and improved cognitive performance..."

Lavender essential oil has a calming scent which makes it a great tonic for nerve and anxiety issues. Therefore, it can also be very helpful in treating migraines, headaches, depression, nervous tension and emotional stress. The refreshing aroma removes nervous exhaustion and restlessness while also increasing mental activity. Lavender has so many other health benefits as well, as shown below in the picture below. As a side note, you can ingest lavender oil only if it is 100% pure therapeutic grade essential oils.

How to use Lavender Essential Oil:

- Diffuse 5-10 drops or steam vaporize throughout the day. Constant exposure to the vapors alleviates both emotional and physical symptoms of depression.
- Lavender essential oil can be used topically in its undiluted form. You can apply it to your pulse points, temples, or the bottom of your feet. You can also dilute it with a carrier oil and rub it on your skin.
- As a quick fix, put a drop or two in the palm of your hands, rub them together and then cup your hands around the nose and mouth then breathe in deeply.
- It can also be used as a dietary supplement only if you are using 100% pure therapeutic grade oil. You can add a drop to a glass of water and drink it or make a Lavender Lemonade. See recipe below:

How To Make Lavender Lemonade To Get Rid Of Headaches and Anxiety

Pure natural honey — 1 cup

Clean drinking water — 12 cups

Lavender essential oil — 1 drop

Organic lemon juice — 6 lemons

www.LoveThisPic.com

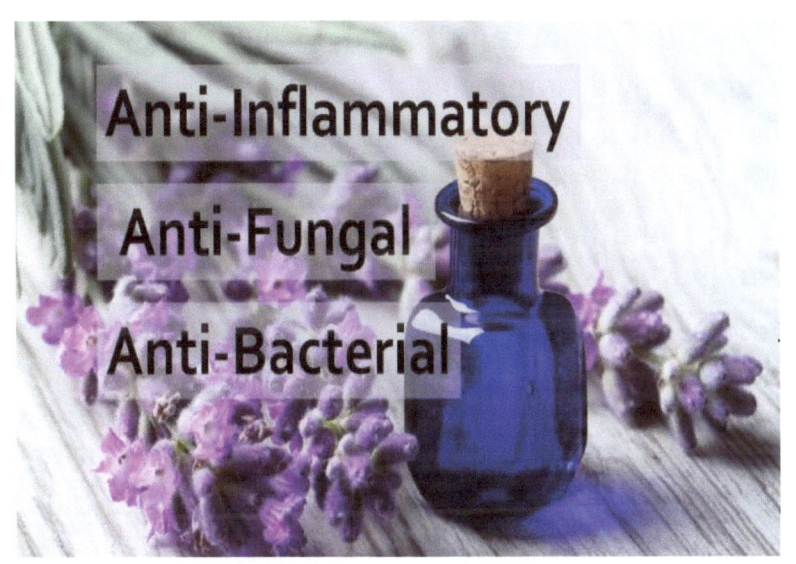

Chapter 4

Bergamot Essential Oil

Bergamot essential oil is a great antidepressant because it is very stimulating. Bergamot can create a feeling of joy, freshness and energy by improving the circulation of your blood. I read an article by Dr. Axe that stated, a 2011 study done in Thailand found that bergamot lowered the anxiety response in rats. Another study found that applying a blended oil that includes bergamot to participants helps treat depression.

You do not have to use toxic antidepressant drugs to fight depression because it has been found they only make matters worse. You can treat depression naturally with essential oils.

Bergamot essential oil is calming, it provides hormonal support, and it's antibacterial and antiseptic. Its fragrant influence relieves anxiety and has the ability to uplift your mood.

Bergamot is known to be used for treating agitation, depression, anxiety, intestinal parasites, insomnia, and viral infections (herpes cold sores).

How to use Bergamot Essential Oil:

- Diffuse
- Take as a dietary supplement
- Dilute 1 part essential oil with 1 part V-6 Vegetable Oil Complex or other pure vegetable oil; apply 1-2 drops on location.
- Apply on Chakras and/or Vita Flex points

- Inhale directly from the bottle

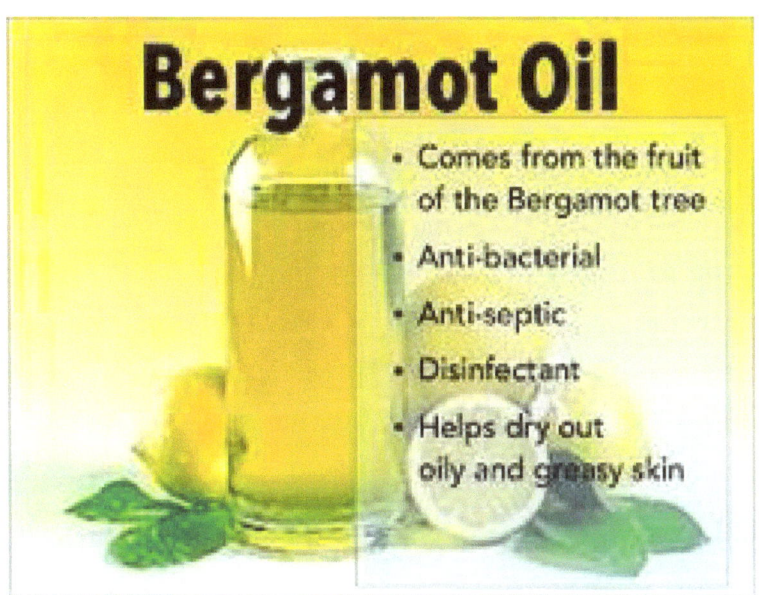

Chapter 5

Roman Chamomile

Inhale directly from the bottle Chamomile is one of the best medicinal herbs for fighting stress and promoting relaxation. Chamomile helps with supporting a healthy mental state by providing qualities that soothe your emotions.

According to research from Alternative Therapies in Health and Medicine and Pharmacognosy Review, inhaling chamomile vapors using chamomile essential oil is often recommended as a natural remedy for anxiety and general depression.

Roman Chamomile is a relaxant, antispasmodic, anti-inflammatory, antiparisitic, antibacterial and antiparasitic. It can be used to relieve restlessness, anxiety, ADHD, depression, insomnia and stress.

Its fragrant influence minimizes anxicty, irrability and nervousness. Because it is calming and relaxing, it can combat depression, insomnia and stress. It may also dispel anger, stabilize the emotions and help to release emotions that are linked to the past.

How to use Roman Chamomile Essential Oil:

- Apply 1-2 drops on location, ankles and wrists.
- Apply on Chakras and/or Vita Flex points
- Diffuse
- Take as a dietary supplement

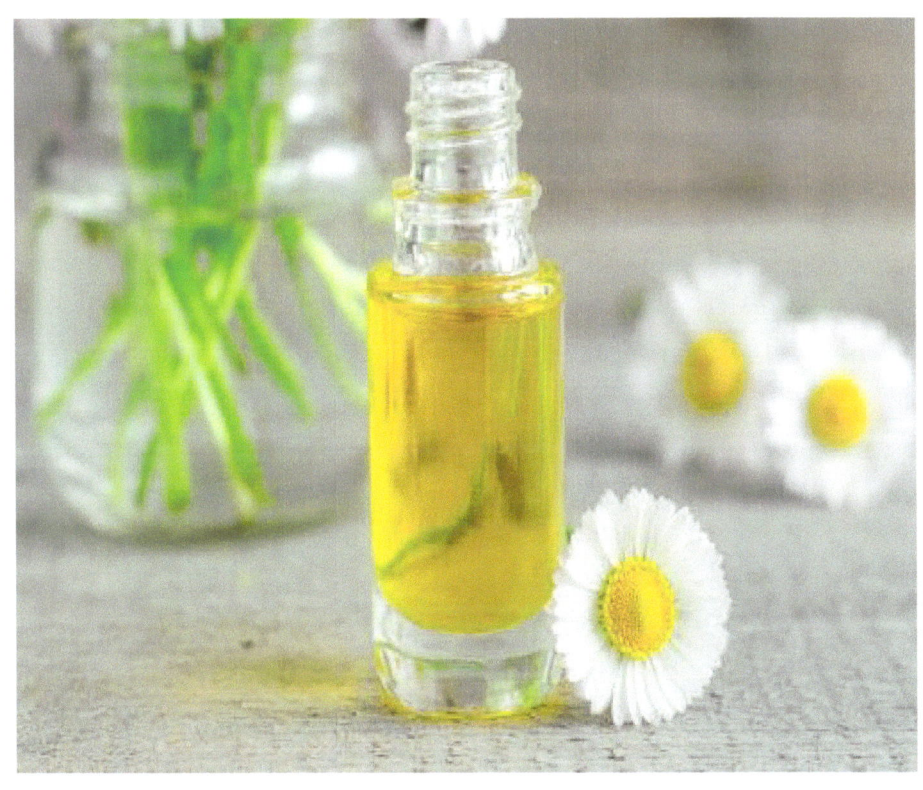

Chapter 6

Ylang Ylang Essential Oil

Last but definitely not least is the oil with the funny name, Ylang Ylang, which means "flower of flowers". It is a beautiful flower native to Madagascar, Ecuador. This oil has amazing benefits for helping you to stave off depression and negative emotions that are associated with depression. Simply inhaling ylang ylang can have immediate positive effects on your mood and act like a mild remedy for depression. Research shows that it can help release negative emotions such as anger, low self-esteem and even jealousy.

Ylang Ylang is also used for cardiac arrhythmia, cardiac problems, anxiety, hypertension, depression, hair loss and intestinal problems. The fragrant influence of ylang ylang balances male-female energies, enhances spiritual attunement, combats anger, combats low self –esteem, increases focus of thoughts, filters out negative energy, restores confidence and peace.

Ylang Ylang works because of its mild sedative like effects which lower stress responses helping you to relax. When you diffuse the oil in your home or massage it into your skin, it enhances your self-confidence, mood and self-love.

How to use Ylang Ylang Essential Oil:

- Diffuse
- Take as a dietary supplement

- Dilute 1 part essential oil with 1 part V-6 Vegetable Oil Complex or other pure vegetable oil; apply 1-2 drops on location.
- Apply on Chakras and/or Vita Flex points
- Inhale directly from the bottle

Ylang Ylang

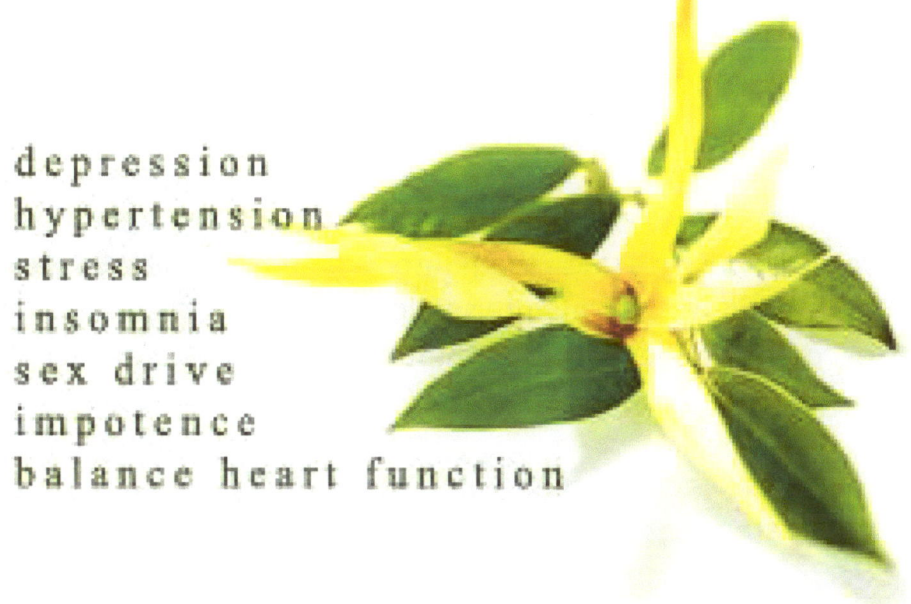

depression
hypertension
stress
insomnia
sex drive
impotence
balance heart function

Chapter 7

Rose Essential Oil

Who can smell a rose and not feel better. Its beautiful fragrance is intoxicating and aphrodisiac-like. It helps to bring balance and harmony, allowing one to overcome insecurities. The effect of rose on the heart brings good feelings which calms and uplifts the spirit.

Rose essential oil has been used for hypertension, heart strengthening, anxiety, viral infections and skin conditions.

According to an article that I read from Dr Josh Axe, the Journal of Complementary Therapies in Clinical Practice recently published a study that stated:

"With a subject group of 28 postpartum women, the researchers separated them into two groups: one who would be treated with 15-minute sessions of a 2.5 percent solution of rose/lavender oil aromatherapy twice a week for four weeks, and a control group.

Their results were quite remarkable. Not only was it discovered that the women experienced a significant decrease in postnatal depression scores, they also reported marked improvement in general anxiety disorder!"

Rose essential oil has the highest frequency or energy out of all the oils mentioned in this book. Its frequency is 320 MHZ! Why is this important, you may ask? Because a healthy body, from head to foot, typically has a **frequency** ranging from 62 to 78 MHz, while disease begins at 57 MHz. Therefore, the higher the frequency or LIFE energy you have the more LIFE you have and the less likely you are to become sick or dis-eased!

How to use Rose Essential Oil:

- Diffuse
- Apply 2-4 drops on location
- Inhale directly from the bottle
- Apply on Chakras and/or Vita Flex points

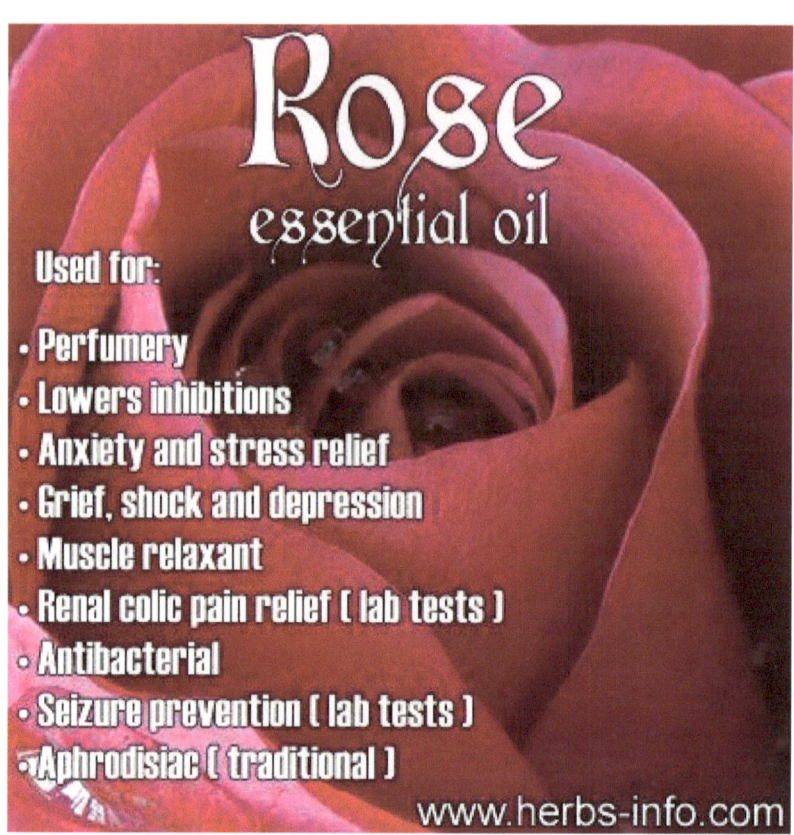

Rose
essential oil

Used for:

- Perfumery
- Lowers inhibitions
- Anxiety and stress relief
- Grief, shock and depression
- Muscle relaxant
- Renal colic pain relief (lab tests)
- Antibacterial
- Seizure prevention (lab tests)
- Aphrodisiac (traditional)

www.herbs-info.com

Photo Credit: herbs-info.com

Closing Remarks

In closing, essential oils are powerful and healing to the body, mind and spirit. They treat the whole person. Essential oils are Life Essences of a plant and are the oldest known medicinal that have absolutely no side effects. Allah (God) gave us everything that we need here on earth to heal ourselves of any condition. We must return to our natural state by turning back to the earth. We came from the earth and so do our solutions. The universe was created to serve MAN! The Original Man, that is!

We Want to Hear From You

If this book has help you in any way to make a healthier lifestyle choice, DeNise would love to hear from you.

Leave a review on Amazon.com

To schedule a consultation with DeNise:

Go to www.denisemuhammad.com

To purchase the essential oils mentioned in this book go to my website: bit.ly/deniseroils

Follow DeNise on Social Media

Facebook & Instagram: DeNise Renee Muhammad

Periscope & Twitter: @DeNiseSelfCare